HCG DIET

Step-By-Step Guide With Easy and
Delicious Recipes for the Hcg Diet and
30-Day Weight Loss Plans for Beginners

By   BETTY   CLARK

Disclaimer Notice

Please note the information contained within this document is for educational and entertainment purposes only. All effort has been executed to present accurate, up to date, and reliable, complete information. No warranties of any kind are declared or implied. Readers acknowledge that the author is not engaging in the rendering of legal, financial, medical or professional advice. The content within this book has been derived from various sources. Please consult a licensed professional before attempting any techniques outlined in this book.

By reading this document, the reader agrees that under no circumstances is the author responsible for any losses, direct or indirect, which are incurred as a result of the use of information contained within this document, including, but not limited to, — errors, omissions, or inaccuracies.

Table of contents

Chapter 1: Introduction

If you are looking to lose weight fast to improve your health then the HCG diet is the best option for your needs. Dieters have been able to lose half a pound or more every day with no negative side effects while on the HCG diet. It's not always the easiest diet to follow, but it's the one that will give you results fast.

This guide will spend some time exploring the HCG diet. You will learn everything that is required to successfully start this diet program. We will talk about what the HCG diet is, the benefits of this diet, the different stages of this diet, what to do if you feel hungry on this diet and also whether you should use the injections or drops on this diet plan. We will finish the guide with some simple HCG approved recipes and a diet calendar that will make the HCG diet much easier to follow and see results.

If you are looking for an easy way to lose weight quickly and efficiently, you can't go wrong with the HCG diet.

Today, many people are still looking for the HCG diet to help them lose weight and feel better. It is sometimes still difficult to get the HCG needed for this diet program without going to a weight loss clinic, but many people don't believe they need medical intervention to do so. Despite some of the challenges of getting HCG, it appears that Dr. Simeons research from the 1950s is still prevalent and helpful for weight loss today.

What is the HCG diet?

There are many diet and weight loss programs that you can choose from. Some of them promise to be the miracle cure you need to start feeling better than ever, but not all of them can deliver on that promise. With all the options available, it can be difficult to know which one can actually provide you with the right results.

While on the HCG diet, you will be limited to around 500 calories each day for a total of three to six weeks. Some people who have a lot of weight to lose may follow the diet for a little longer or may do a few different cycles of the diet to help them. You also need to take oral drops or HCG hormone shots during this time to help with weight loss.

At this time, the FDA has not approved the HCG diet or the injections you need to do. This hasn't stopped many people from trying and enjoying the results. Shots are not considered illegal, as long as you can find a health care provider to give them to you as HCG is approved to help with fertility issues.

When you are on an HCG diet, you will not be allowed to eat a lot. The diet allows you to have two main meals during the day, a lunch and a dinner. Each meal must include a fruit, a bread, a vegetable and a protein. You can choose to divide your meals into snacks or even have breakfast, but remember that you can only get up to 500 calories a day with this diet plan.

If you follow this diet, you will find that the amount of effort you have to put in can be difficult. 500 calories a day is not that easy and can be really uncomfortable to do. Considering you have to stick to the 500 calories for a few weeks, it can also be dangerous for you. It is virtually impossible to achieve the nutritional needs your body requires with so many calories. But for those desperate to lose weight to improve their overall health, this may be the best option to help you.

For those on other special diets, such as a vegetarian or vegan diet, this will be a little more difficult to follow.

The HCG diet can be difficult for some people to follow. You really need to limit how much you are eating for a few months and you need to take daily injections of the HCG hormone to see results. For those who have tried everything and are not getting the desired results, this may be the best option to help them lose weight.

How does the HCG diet work?

If you are interested in starting the HCG diet, there are four different stages you will go through. Understanding these steps will help you better follow the HCG diet and get the results you are looking for. The different stages you need to follow with the HCG diet include:

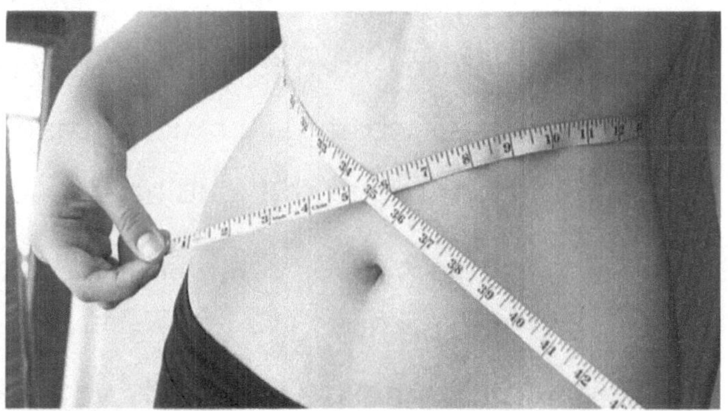

Phase 1

The first phase of this diet plan is known as the loading phase. This was not originally included in the HCG diet, but was added later when Kevin Trudeau reintroduced this diet. During this two day period, you will consume high calorie foods until you are satisfied. You shouldn't overeat and stretch too much, but eat until you feel satisfied and full.

The point is to help satisfy some of the addictions and food cravings you may have during the other periods of this diet plan. It has been shown that those who do not add this phase to their diet plan before entering phase two will often have stronger cravings than those who go through the loading phase.

To do this phase, you will start taking HCG on the first day of phase one. When it comes to the foods you want to eat, make sure you eat the ones you usually crave so that you can get rid of temptation. Also, choose more calorie foods so that you can build up the fat stores in your body early.

You can basically choose any day you want to start the upload phase. However, it is best not to start it near the menstrual cycle. Some people also choose to use three days of load instead of two days. You should choose the amount of time that you think is best for your needs.

Phase 2

The second phase will be one of the most challenging parts of the HCG diet. This is the weight loss phase, where rapid weight loss will occur at a steady pace. This part will last three to six weeks depending on how much weight you need to lose. During this second phase, the dieter will take the HCG injection every day and then have to follow a low calorie diet. If you follow exactly this, you will see weight loss every day when you weigh yourself.

So, the first thing you will do each day when you enter phase two is to take the HCG tablets, drops or injections. You will be able to adjust the amount of HCG you are taking to suit your personal needs, but more often than not the dosage isn't all that important. If you always feel hungry on this diet, you may want to increase the dosage a bit.

During phase two, you will need to be on a diet with less than 500 calories per day. Some individuals find that they can still lose weight by eating more than 500 calories, but to see the best results, you'll stick to that calorie quota. The HCG hormone will help you maintain this amount of calories without feeling deprived.

During this day, you can also implement an apple day. To make an apple day, you need to start at noon one day and finish at noon the other day. The purpose of these days is to address the problem of water retention and it can help you if you see a stalemate in your weight loss. During this day, you can eat up to six apples, any type is fine, and reduce your water intake. This will help you avoid cravings and get you back on track.

You will need to stay in phase 2 for up to six weeks. Some people have been successful for a little longer, and it often depends on how much weight you need to lose and how fast you want to lose it. However, there is limited success that goes beyond six weeks. It is often best to cycle this phase, take a break, and then go back and do another six weeks at a different time if you still need to lose weight.

Phase 3

Phase three is known as the stabilization phase of this diet. This phase will occur when the dieter has finished the second phase and is no longer taking the hormone HCG. This will usually last for about three weeks. During this part, you will slowly add more calories and more foods to your menu. You need to add foods slowly, one or two at a time, so that you can get used to the food and don't overdo it after the calorie-restricted diet.

Phase three should last around three weeks. However, if you end up gaining more than two pounds in that three week period, there are some special steps you need to take and you will start the three weeks again. The third phase is meant to help you get back to eating more calories, without overdoing it and eating the bad foods you did before. You will stay in this phase until you can keep your weight stabilized for a full three weeks.

Phase 4

The final stage is the maintenance stage. Here you will work to maintain the weight loss you saw in the other stages and keep it forever. This phase is meant to last for the rest of your life (until you want to do another cycle). The HCG plan should help you learn to stick to the maintenance phase without too much trouble because you will learn how to avoid unhealthy sugars and fats, eat only when you are hungry, learn balance and eat only when you are really hungry. It is about learning to listen to your body. If you have been successful during the other phases of the HCG diet, this shouldn't be too difficult to follow.

All stages of the HCG diet are important in helping you see the weight loss you are looking for. Make sure you follow each one right and you will be sure to see results in no time.

Chapter 2: Benefits of the HCG diet

Before starting any type of diet, it is important to know the benefits of its use. The HCG diet can be difficult to use. You need to be on a very low-calorie diet for about six weeks, sticking to 500 calories or less. And you also need to have an injection or drops of HCG every day for about eight weeks while on a diet. Maintaining both of these parts can take a lot of time and dedication, and you need to be ready to move forward to see results.

The good news is that there are many benefits to using the HCG diet. The first benefit is that when you take the HCG hormone, it helps you not feel as hungry as before. This makes it much easier to stick to the 500 calories needed for drastic weight loss. If you've ever tried to limit calories in the past, you know how difficult it can be. Thinking of cutting calories by up to 500 over the course of a few months may seem impossible. But with the help of the HCG hormone, you are not only signaling the body to burn more fat, but you are also helping to limit cravings and can actually feel full on such a low calorie diet.

The main benefit you will get from the HCG diet is that you will lose a lot of weight. Once you have entered the second phase, it is possible to lose a pound or more per day. The results will depend on how much weight you need to lose in the first place. Those who just need to lose a few pounds will find that they don't lose a lot of weight. But those who have a lot of weight to lose may be able to lose more than half a pound every day.

This diet plan, with the help of the HCG hormone, can also help you have enough energy to get things done throughout the day. With a traditional low calorie diet plan, you will feel sluggish and tired all the time. You may be able to keep calories restricted for some time, but your body will feel it, and because you're so tired, you'll want to get back to your normal diet in no time. With the help of the HCG hormone, you can maintain your energy reserves and feel good all the time.

Of course, when you are losing weight on this diet plan, there are a whole host of other benefits that you can enjoy at the same time. When you lose weight, you can help protect your heart health, lower cholesterol levels, reduce stress, lower blood pressure, improve your mental functioning, and so much more. And this diet allows you to reap these great health benefits in no time without feeling deprived.

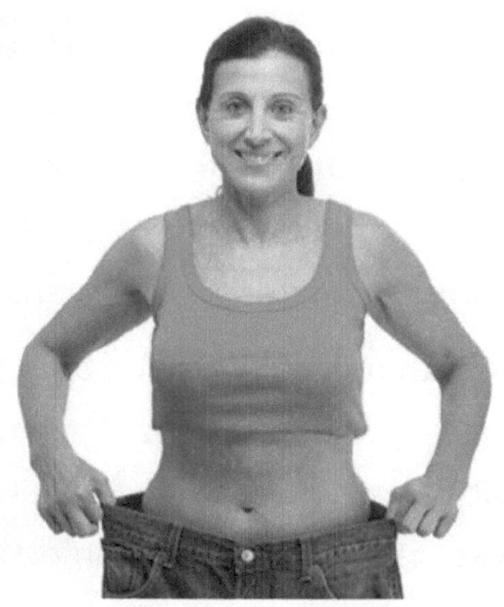

When you are looking for a diet plan that will help you lose weight quickly and effectively so you can get your health back on track, then the HCG diet is the one for you.

What can you expect?

Each person who decides to follow the HCG diet has different expectations of what will happen. This diet plan is different than what you can find when it comes to losing weight. It has been around for some time now, but you have to rely on consuming very few calories and taking injections of the HCG hormone, which is not even recommended on other diet plans.

The first thing you will have to get used to is getting the injections. This might be a little scary for some people who are just starting out. These injections are relatively safe and have been used in a medical setting to help treat infertility problems in women. Most people on the HCG diet have been able to self-administer these injections in no time with limited problems. If you are really worried about taking these injections, there are other methods of taking these hormones, including drops, topical options, and more.

Sometimes people will find that the 500 calories will be too difficult for them to manage. This is a very limited amount of food and for those dealing with low blood sugar or other health problems, limiting yourself so much can be scary. However, thanks to the HCG hormone you are taking, you won't feel hungry like when you limit these calories on your own. In many cases, you will be able to limit calories and feel good.

If you find calories are a little too restrictive, there are many who have upped them a bit to feel better. This is usually reserved for those who train a lot and who need some extra nutrients in their diet to stay healthy. Usually, you should keep it close to 500 calories; most people will choose to eat 600 or 700 calories instead.

The biggest change you will see when following this diet plan is the rate at which you can see weight and fat loss. There are a few factors that come into play as to how much weight you will be able to lose during this diet program.

The amount you need to lose when starting this diet will greatly affect your weight loss. If you have a lot of weight to lose, you will see it drop quickly at the start of this diet plan. It will level out the longer you are on this diet plan. Many people claim that they can lose a pound or more every day when following this diet plan.

Remember this is not a full-time or permanent diet plan. Other plans allow you to at least maintain them until you lose all the weight you need or want.

However, this is not recommended when following the HCG diet. If you have a significant amount of weight to lose, it's best to do six weeks on the HCG diet and then six weeks off and then go back and forth. This makes it a little easier to stick to the calories and ensures that you won't get stuck with this diet plan.

Most people find it safe to follow this diet plan. You should learn to listen to your body while on a diet. If you feel that you are losing weight too fast or that your body cannot handle this low calorie content, then it may be time to add more calories or stop the diet.

The HCG diet is really effective in helping you lose a lot of weight fast, but it's a little different than some of the other diet plans you may have tried in the past. Understanding what will happen while you are on this diet plan can make it easier to stick to this diet plan for your weight loss success.

Hence, this diet is working to limit the daily calorie intake. Now, let's do some math. But before we start, we need to know that a kilo of fat is worth 3,500 kcal or 1 kg is worth 7,700 kcal.

The daily calorie requirement for a woman is 2,000 kcal and 2,500 kcal for a man.

So now we can say that to lose half a kilo of fat we need to burn 3,500 kcal. In this diet we only eat 500 kcal of the 2,000 kcal we need to maintain our weight. So that's 1,500 kcal that we burn automatically. So we need 2.3 days to lose half a kilo if we eat 500 kcal every day.

This is the math: 3,500 / 1,500 = 2.33

So, in one day you will see a weight loss of 0.43lbs (1500kcal / 3500kcal). If you lose more than that, you are burning more than 2,000 calories per day.

This could be due to increased physical activity, age and metabolic rate.

Injections or drops?

When you are ready to start the HCG diet, you will have to choose whether you want to use the injections or the drops to get the hormones into your body. There are some benefits and some downsides to using them and sometimes it will depend on what you are most comfortable with, how much money you have to spend and your lifestyle. The HCG diet is tough enough, so if it's easier for you to take the drops or the idea of having an injection every day scares you, then stick with the drops. There are some people who say that the only effective way to do this diet plan. But when you add the HCG hormone with a calorie restricted diet, you are sure to see the weight loss you desire.

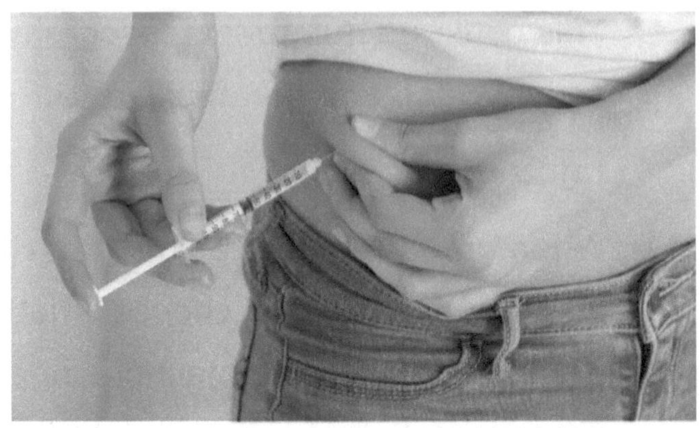

HCG injections

When it comes to getting HCG injections, you can only get them by prescription. Whether you get them from your local pharmacy or are following this diet with help from your doctor, getting the supplies can be really easy. If not, you will need to procure your supplies online. These prescriptions can be expensive, sometimes costing more than $ 400 or more, and you may even need to visit your doctor every week. Some dieters order their supplies online to save some money.

When you decide to order your HCG hormone online, make sure you get the right amount and can mix the solution yourself. Some people don't have a problem with this, but it can make others nervous, so keep that in mind. You also need to worry about how safe it is to order your HCG online. Most pharmacies offering this hormone will be reliable and offer you a good product, you must always be careful where you are ordering your supplies from.

There are also some side effects that come with the use of HCG injections. Most of these side effects will be caused by the needle. You may find bruising and irritation from the injection site, and others find that giving the injections can be painful. If these side effects are making you nervous or you feel that you will not be able to perform these injections on your own, it might be a good idea to look into the HCG drops.

HCG drops

You can also choose to do the drops too. This is a good option for those who need to save money on this diet plan or if you are nervous about using needles for injections. You can take the drops sublingually or put them under the tongue to help them absorb better. These drops will be mixed in your home, which is important because HCG degrades quickly and you need to put them in the fridge right away. You can get these drops from your pharmacy or doctor, or you can find them through an online company.

These drops usually cost less than injections, which makes them a great option for most people. However, there are many people who think these drops are more of a nuisance than injections. You are not allowed to drink or eat anything for half an hour after taking the drops, and this can be a problem for some. And if these drops are not absorbed properly, you may have problems with hunger and eat more calories than the HCG diet allows.

When it comes to doing it, it often depends on your personal goals and what works best for your needs when choosing whether to go with the injections or the drops. You can choose based on what you are comfortable with, the budget you have to spend on this diet, and how easy it is for you to get supplies. Both can be effective, especially when combined with a low calorie diet, in helping you lose a lot of weight.

Chapter 3: When hunger strikes

With the HCG diet, you are drastically limiting the amount of calories you are consuming. You can only eat 500 calories during the day and this can be difficult. At some point, you will likely experience hunger while following this diet plan. However, you should note that these hunger pains will subside after about five days on the diet, as long as you take the hormone correctly and eat the right foods.

Hunger often subsides after this period of time as your body will begin to harness the excess fat in your body and use those calories to give you the energy you need. This is where fat and weight loss will come into play, especially once you get into the ketosis process. You simply have to be able to get through those few days of starvation to see the amazing results.

The good news for dieters is that while they may feel hungrier during days five to seven on HCG, they will also see the greatest weight loss during that time. So while you might get a little frustrated during this time because you are feeling so hungry, you will get the reward of losing weight every day. This can be a powerful motivator when it comes to staying on the diet plan and keeping it up to the end.

However, ignoring those hunger pains can be a big challenge during the first week of the HCG diet. You need to keep calories down to 500 (or nearly so) if you want to be able to actually lose the promised weight. There are three main steps you can take to make it easier to overcome these hunger pains.

These three steps include:

Upload properly

To some people, the loading phase may seem like it goes against your weight loss goals. Why should you spend time giving in to your cravings and eating lots of calories when you want to lose weight? But the loading phase of the HCG diet is as important as any other. First, it helps provide the body with an immediate calorie reserve, enough to help you last days three, four, and five. It also helps you metabolize fat better because you have increased the amount of fat you are consuming.

During the loading phase, it is best to load as much fat as possible. Carbohydrates can be fine too, but most of your focus has to be on fat. This helps you have excess stores in your body when it's time to start the HCG diet and can make weight loss a lot easier. You may have some unhealthy fats during this time, but for those who are concerned, go with healthier fats like nuts, avocados, and salmon to help you out.

Prepare food in advance

Sometimes the biggest problem with this diet is that you are tempted to eat more than you should. You get hungry and then you start snacking as you prepare meals. Or you find that there is nothing prepared in the house, so you go out to eat and spoil all your efforts.

One way to avoid this problem is to prepare meals in advance. Often, it's all about convenience when it comes to which foods to consume with your diet. Finding out what foods are allowed on the HCG diet and then preparing them in advance makes our life easier. We will eat and continue with these foods because they are already available to eat and are cheaper than doing something else or going out to eat.

Cheat correctly

For the most part, you should stick to the 500 calories if you want to see all the weight loss promised by this diet plan. However, for some people, the 500 calories won't be enough. In some cases, you may want to consider adding a few extra calories. You still need to choose foods that are approved on the HCG diet. The best option to go with are foods that are not only allowed on the HCG diet, but those that are full of nutrients and can really fill you up. Eat lots of them and you'll be less likely to be hungry.

There are several foods that you can use as a cheat on the HCG diet. If you find that your calories are not enough when you limit yourself to 500, it's okay to eat as many as you want as long as you eat slowly and don't eat them simply because you're bored.

Some of the foods that you can consider as cheating foods include:

Green vegetables: Green vegetables are usually good for eating more on the HCG diet. Just make sure you don't eat cucumbers or anything else that has seeds in them as these will contain more carbohydrates than other options.

Chicken Broth: These cubes or bags usually contain less than 30 calories each, but adding some to the water and sipping can be really filling. Some people are worried about all the extra sodium. But doing it occasionally won't cause more of a problem.

Dried meat: If you include dried meat in your diet, make sure you are getting a good type with a lot of protein in it. Jerky has a good protein, fat, and carbohydrate ratio, so it's the perfect snack. Adding a few grams between meals and perhaps adding a few stalks of celery can help you feel less hungry as you lose weight.

There will be times when you will feel hungry on the HCG diet, mainly because you are cutting calories a bit. The good news is that your body will soon tap into the excess fat stores within and you will see a large amount of fat and weight loss in no time. Add the HCG hormone and you will be able to see weight loss, without much hunger, in no time.

Another thing the hormone does is make you feel full.

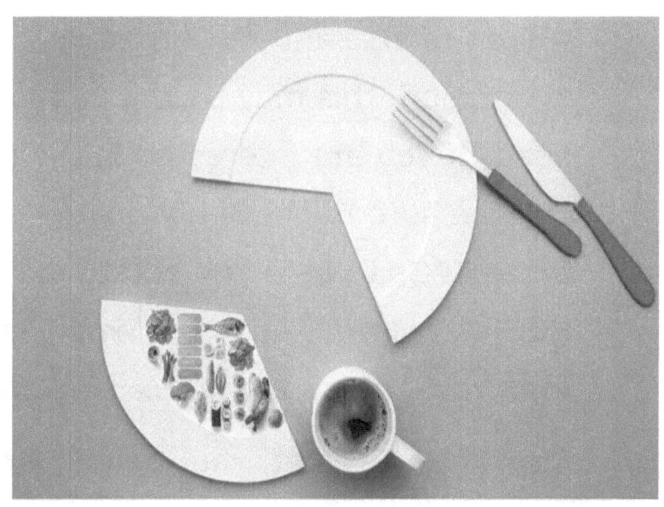

Chapter 4: Frequently Asked Questions About the HCG Diet

Starting the HCG diet can be difficult. You have to be careful how many calories you eat each day to keep it low. You also need to take a few injections or a few drops if you want to see results. All of this must come together to see the weight loss that has been promised to you. The good news is that if you can follow all the steps, you can easily lose one or more pounds every day. For those who have a lot of weight to lose and have tried everything, this may be the diet you need. If you are interested in the HCG diet, be sure to check out some of these FAQs to help you determine if the HCG diet is right for you. ***Will I regain lost body mass after the HCG diet?***

After the HCG diet, your benefit isn't just limited to body mass loss. Former HCG dieters also reported a change in hunger and an innate course of altered eating behavior and metabolic rate.

They likewise reported this through a perfect situation aimed at easily transitioning into a suitable relationship with food. With all these changes, as well as experiences, the HCG diet represents the ideal opportunity to adopt a healthy lifestyle and preserve body mass.

There really is no basis for regaining the lost pounds, as long as you've managed to replace any previous negative eating and sedentary lifestyle routines with fresh, healthy views on diet and training.

Most post-HCG dieters have found that the minimum amount of daily activity is enough to maintain their HCG goal on weight loss. A minimal amount of training is suggested not only for maintaining body mass, but also for extra health values. Recommended activities include 20-minute cardio exercise, yoga, or any other activity that you enjoy and that allows your cardiovascular system to move. Through the hypothalamus, you can restore your metabolic rate to reflect these changes and allow yourself to consume moderately, without feeling the need or temptation to overdo it.

Is HCG safe for males too?

The HCG hormone is present in men
innately. It is actually present in every
tissue of all human beings, male or
female, and logically pregnant or not
for females. The quantity simply
escalates in pregnant women.
Additionally, millions of men have used
the HCG regimen to shed weight in a
positive way.

What is the maximum weight I can lose using the HCG diet?

A census was conducted which included
over 7,000 dieters using HCG. Relapses
showed an average loss of two pounds
each day. Most of these people on a
program reported losing half a pound
per day.

However, it remains important that all
dissimilar results may differ based on
individual encounters. The results could
be affected by an individual's unique
personal body vibrations, their menu,

and the amount of action while following the standard.

Who is considered the correct candidate for HCG diet injections?

The mass of then healthy, but severely obese men, as well as women, can become optimal patients aiming to use HCG diet drops and shots to lose weight. People are advised to see a doctor for an interview before starting the HCG diet.

It is also suggested that people who choose this as their diet, follow the instructions of a doctor or a qualified expert accordingly for the correct application of the HCG protocol.

What is HCG?

HCG, or human chorionic gonadotropin, is a hormone that is already produced in small quantities in women and men. Pregnant women often produce it in larger quantities. HCG has the task of influencing the functioning of the metabolism by stimulating the hypothalamus. The HCG hormone has traditionally been used in medicine to help with infertility problems in women and with low testosterone levels in men.

The idea of HCG in this diet plan is to speed up your metabolism so that you can lose weight even faster. You would take the HCG hormone in the form of drops or an injection, to help with weight loss. When you combine it with a calorie restricted diet, you will be able to see a lot of weight loss in a short amount of time.

Is It Legal To Use HCG For Weight Loss?

It is legal to use HCG for weight loss. The FDA does not technically approve the 500 calorie diet that comes with the HCG diet, but it is legal to use HCG. In fact, HCG is currently used as a way to treat infertility in women, and many doctors are okay with prescribing it as a weight loss tool. There are also some newer versions of the HCG diet that allow for a higher calorie intake allowed by the FDA.

Who will do well on the HCG diet?

Most overweight, but otherwise healthy patients, be they men or women, can be considered potential patients for using the HCG diet for weight loss. It is best if you take the time to talk to your doctor before starting this diet. This ensures that you have no underlying conditions that could be affected when following this diet plan.

Are there any side effects to the drops or injections?

There are some side effects of following the HCG diet and using both drops and injections. However, very few patients ever report any of these side effects. When the HCG hormone is used as a fertility treatment, the larger amount needed for that treatment can sometimes cause pregnancy symptoms and occasional headaches.

However, it is important to note that when following the HCG diet, you will be taking a much lower dosage of HCG than is used in fertility treatments. Sometimes the patient will experience a little hunger, dizziness and hunger. It is often considered the fault of the protocol and the lack of calories you are eating, which will cause these problems.

How Much Can I Lose With This Diet Plan?

The amount you can lose on this diet program varies based on a number of factors. Your age, weight, metabolism, and whether you are a boy or a girl can all determine how much weight you can lose when you follow the HCG diet.

There was a recent survey conducted that included more than 7,000 people who followed the HCG diet. The results showed that on average, the participants lost half a kilo to half a kilo each day. There were also some participants who lost up to 3 pounds in one day. These are the average results of the diet plan and each person will see different results when following the HCG diet. As long as you learn your body chemistry so that you can make adjustments if necessary, you will be able to lose weight with this diet plan.

Is it safe for men to take HCG?

The HCG hormone is actually found in men naturally. While you will find HCG in the highest concentrations in pregnant women, it is produced in a decent amount in anyone. This means that there are men who also have the HCG hormone naturally. In fact, there are millions of men who are going to use the HCG diet to help them lose weight without much hassle.

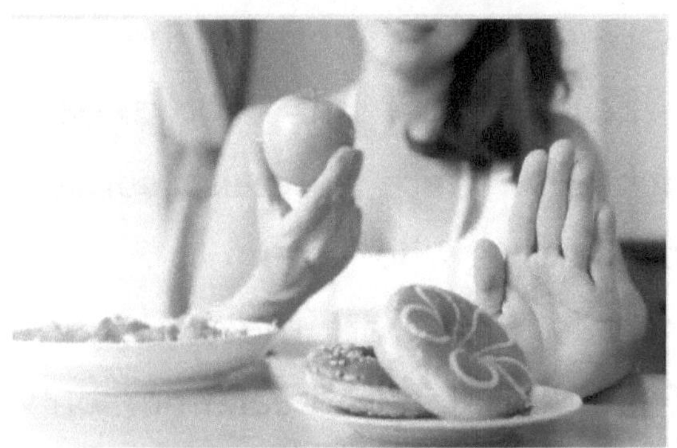

Where do I get the injections or the drops?

There are several places where you can get the injections or the drops. If you are working with a health care practitioner to follow this diet, you will be able to get the HCG hormone from them. This is a good way to get the HCG hormone because you know it will be safe and you won't have to do a lot of research about it. If you want to cut costs a little or are following this diet without the supervision of a doctor or other health care professional, you can choose to buy the drops or injections online and mix the solution yourself.

Is it really healthy to lose so much weight every day?

When you follow the HCG diet, you will see a lot of weight loss in a short amount of time. This diet plan is successful in giving you rapid weight loss while stimulating the body to maintain lean muscle mass over the long term. Since your weight loss will come directly from unhealthy fats, it will not strip the body of the muscles that are in the body. When you add all the healthy foods you will learn to cook, you will still be able to lose weight (while still nourishing the body at the same time. Eventually, you will end up eating healthier when you are done than you were at the beginning.

Are HCG injections painful?

The injections you will receive of HCG to help with weight loss will be administered through a small and very fine needle. Also, the HCG hormone will be administered to a not so sensitive area. Most dieters report that injections aren't all that painful. For those who are concerned that these injections are too painful or that they may not be able to give themselves the injections, you can use the drops instead.

Where do I inject the shots?

The simplest and most comfortable place to inject the HCG hormone is in the stomach. You should be about two inches from the ship. You can also administer these injections in the thigh or back of the arm if this is easier for you.

Will I get hungry on the HCG diet?

There are some dieters who claim to feel hungry when following this diet in the beginning. This is because they are following a low calorie diet to lose weight. But with the help of the HCG hormone and the fat burning that should occur with this diet plan, the hunger shouldn't last long.

Will I regain all the weight when I'm done?

Not only is the HCG diet great for helping you lose weight, it also focuses on helping you change your current eating habits into something that is much healthier for the whole body. If you successfully complete the HCG diet, you will be better equipped to make healthy food choices, rather than eating the junk you made before, and the weight should stay off even when you are done taking the HCG injections or drops.

If you stop your HCG diet and go back to your old eating habits, it is possible that you can regain weight. If you take in too many calories for your body, it will happen no matter what diet you are on. However, the third phase of HCG is meant to help you safely adjust from the weight loss portion of the HCG diet to the maintenance phase and will make it easier for you to keep the weight off.

Chapter 5: HCG approved diet foods

You will really need to watch the foods you are eating when you are in the second phase of the diet plan. The first phase will primarily focus on consuming the foods you crave so that you can eliminate those temptations. The last two stages will build on the second stage, allowing you to eat healthier than you ever imagined possible. But to see the biggest weight loss on this diet, you need to be really aware of what you eat during the second phase. Some of the different foods (as well as the amount of each food) you should consume during this second phase include:

Protein

- You need to take one serving of protein twice a day. Each serving will be approximately 100 grams (3.5 ounces) for each serving. You need to weigh crude protein and make sure no seasonings or other preparations have been made before weighing. Some of the different protein sources you can choose from include:

- Chicken breast

- Beef (make sure you can get it as lean as possible.

- Shrimp

- Crab

- Lobster

- White fish including tilapia, sole, sea bass, flounder, trout, cod and catfish.

- One egg and three egg whites

- 100 grams of cottage cheese

- **Vegetables**

- You also need to take in some vegetables to provide the nutrients your body needs to stay healthy. The serving size is not indicated in this diet plan. The original protocol does not state how large the portion should be or how many portions you should stick to. You can eat them with satisfaction. Some vegetables allowed in this diet plan include:

- Tomatoes

- Spinach

- Radishes

- Onions

- Lettuce

- Fennel

- Cucumber

- Celery

- Cabbage

- Swiss chard

- Asparagus

- **Fruit**

- Some of the fruits you can enjoy on this diet include a handful of strawberries, an orange, half a grapefruit, and an apple.

- **Carbohydrates**

- There are some carbohydrates you can get in the second phase of the HCG diet. However, most

carbohydrates are reduced
because they are so high in
calories. Carbohydrates you can
have include a piece of toast and
a Grissini stick without the oil.

- **Other options**

- Some of the other options you
  can choose from include a lemon
  and some milk each day. Spices
  and herbs are fine as long as you
  read the label and make sure
  there are no fillers, sweeteners,
  sugars or other things inside. You
  should also be cautious about
  using sweeteners in this diet plan,
  not consuming sugar when it is
  not needed.

- As you can see, there are some
  limitations that occur when
  following this diet plan. You can
  only have 500 calories each day
  on this diet plan to see results

and you have to choose from the options listed above. This can make it difficult for some people just starting out, but if you really want to see results with this diet plan, you'll have to stick to the limitations.

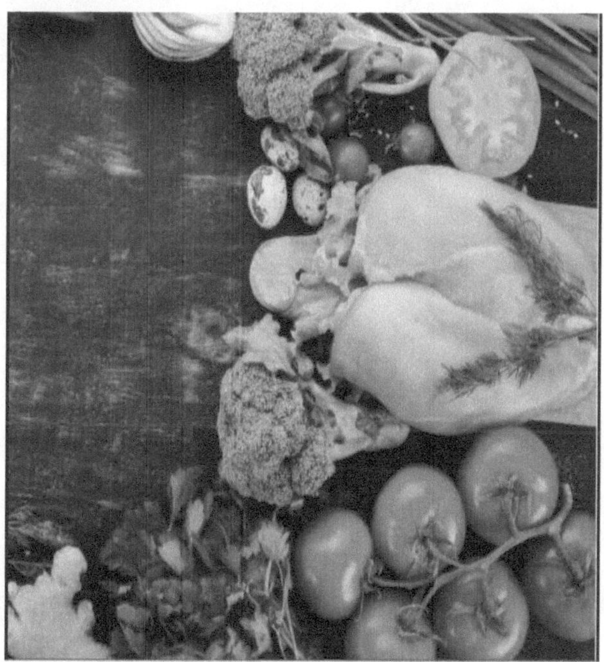

The loading phase

(Days 1 and 2)

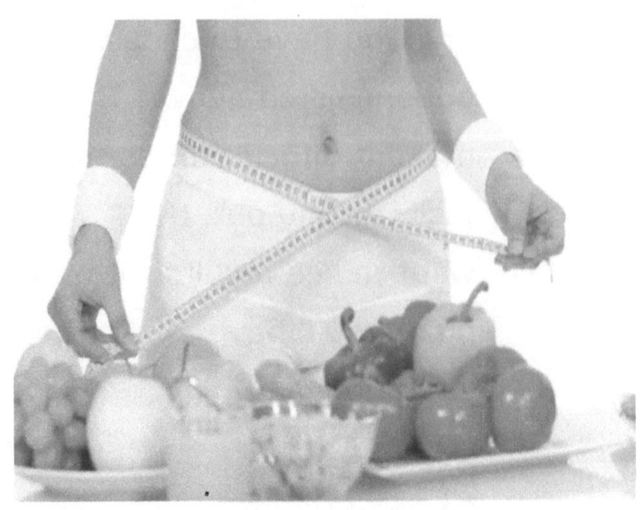

The first phase of the HCG diet program is the "Loading Phase". This step must not be skipped. People who skip the meal plan at this stage are more likely to starve on the third day. Phase 1 prepares the body for the diet. It is during this stage that you start taking HCG. Once the HCG is taken, via HCG injection or HCG drops, you can eat whatever and as much as you want.

The number of times the HCG must be taken depends on the instructions of the HCG. For 2 days, you need to

consume a lot of fatty foods and
starchy foods.

It is recommended to eat the following foods shown below:

- Ice-cream

- Pasta

- Cake

- Candies

- Cookies

- Peanuts

- Olives

- Cheese

- Avocado

- Butter

- Coconut oil

- Flavored Jam

- Cheese cream

- Mayonnaise

- Hamburger

- Rich toppings

- Bagel or other bread

- Mashed potatoes

- Mutton/ Beef

- Extra olive oil

If there are other foods that you crave, you may want to eat those foods as well. On the third day, you will need to move on to the second phase where you start the 500 calorie diet. Phase 1 also recommends that you start drinking more water each day and start engaging in light exercise only.

The maintenance phase

(Days 3 to 23)

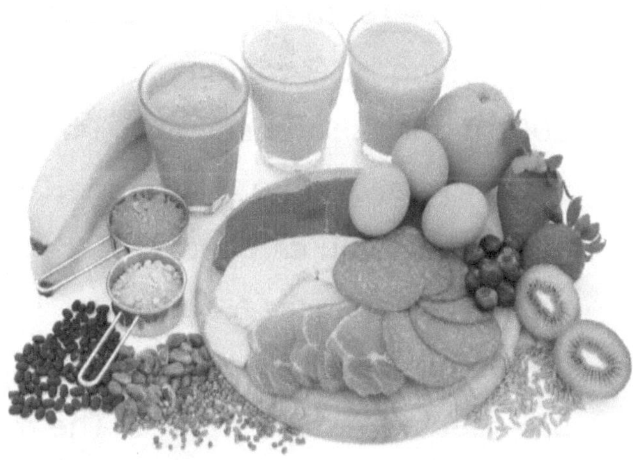

The "Maintenance Phase" is the second phase of the HCG diet plan. This is where the 500 calorie diet begins for a couple of weeks while taking the HCG, either by injection or by drops.

Unlike other diet plans, the HCG diet plan during this phase does not include fats and starches at all. All foods to eat should be measured. Fat or oil cannot be used when cooking a dish. It is recommended that you drink plenty of water at this stage.

On day 24 to 26 of the HCG diet plan, stop taking HCG while continuing the 500 calorie diet these days. Two meals a day are allowed at this stage. For every meal you can eat a toast or any type of breadstick. A portion of 100 grams of meat is allowed for each meal, provided all fat is removed. The meat can be cooked however you like except for frying. The following are the suggested meats to be consumed at this stage:

- Turkey

- Chicken breast

- Pig

- Crab

- Lean beef

- White fish

- Scallops

- Shrimps

You can only have one cup of vegetables per meal. Only one type is allowed per meal. It is not allowed to combine or mix vegetables. Below is the list of recommended vegetables:

- Celery

- Spinach

- Cabbage

- Asparagus

- Broccoli

- Tomatoes

- Onions

- Beets

- Cauliflower

- Cucumber

- Cabbage

- Leeks

- Lettuce

- Brussels sprouts

- Kale

- Dandelion

- Radishes

- Turnips

- Zucchini

- Sweet green and red peppers

- Watercress

- Radishes

> In the second phase, one fruit per meal is allowed. The combination of fruit is also not allowed. Below is the list of fruits you can eat:

- Apple

- Lemon

- Strawberries

- Blackberries

- Blue berries

- Grapefruit

Food intake during breakfast is not allowed. Breakfast should only consist of water, coffee and tea. Stevia is the only sweetener allowed. This is a natural sweetener that can be purchased at health food stores.

The stabilization phase

(Days 27 to 48)

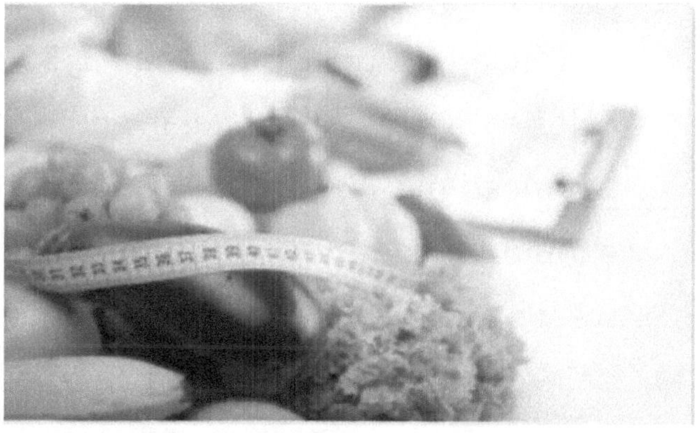

The third phase of the HCG diet program is the "Stabilization Phase". This is also known as the transition phase and the most important of all phases.

This phase is aimed at stabilizing and maintaining the weight. This is the stage where calorie restrictions are reduced. From a very low-calorie diet, you can gradually move to a higher one. As mentioned in the previous chapter of my book, on the last day of taking HCG, you need to keep following the 500 calorie diet rule for another 3 days.

After 3 days, food intake can be increased, but no more than 1,500 calories per day. A regular and balanced diet is allowed. This process should be continued for another 2 to 3 weeks. Small portions or amounts of dairy products and healthy fats, such as avocado, coconut oil, and extra olive oil, can be consumed in the maintenance phase. Continuously avoid eating sugar and starchy foods. This phase is also the "No Sugar, No Starch" phase. Protein intake is the most important during the third phase. Below is the list of foods to avoid during phase 3:

- Rice or Pasta

- Flour Crackers

- Rice or Cereals or Bread or Pasta or Tortilla or White Sugar or Brown Sugar or Maple Sugar /

- Syrup or Powdered

- Sugar or Potatoes or

- Parsnips or Carrots or

- Beans or Legumes

Phase 3 requires you to weigh yourself every morning. Your body weight should not exceed 2 kilos or drop below 2 kilos from your last weight. Your body weight shouldn't change for 4 consecutive days. If your body weight has increased or decreased, increase your protein intake.

Protein is not stored as fat in the body. Having a "Steak Day" is part of the third phase. This is usually done if body weight increases or decreases by 2 pounds.

"Steak Day" is discussed in the next chapters.

The stage of life

(Forever)

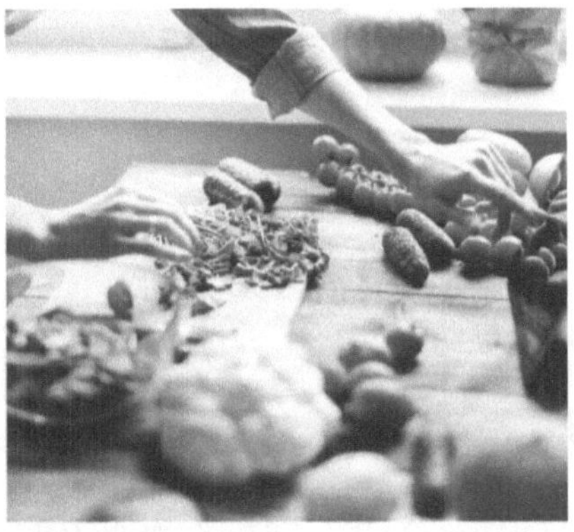

This is the final stage of the HCG diet. This is when food intake normalizes. Sugars and starches can be gradually added to the diet. You will be able to enjoy a healthy and balanced diet and maintain your weight. You will also notice that you are rarely hungry and that you no longer crave the foods you ate.

You can still indulge in your favorite foods from time to time. Being aware of your weight is very important after the HCG diet program. Track your weight on a daily basis. This phase is the extension of the "Stabilization Phase" in which healthy carbohydrates, sugar and starch are slowly added to your daily diet.

If you gain weight, there is no need to panic. You simply have to do the "Steak Day" diet program. It will reduce your weight overnight. After the 500 calorie diet plan, always remember to know your limit. Stay away or avoid eating overly processed foods. This is also the time when you can engage in heavy exercise. It can help keep your figure slim.

Steak day

"Steak Day" is only performed if your weight has increased or decreased by 2 pounds in 4 consecutive days during the third phase of the HCG diet program. The main goal of eating a large serving of steak is to feed the body with protein. The steak protein releases the water weight that is not drained from the body and can eliminate toxins.

This is an effective technique, according to Dr. Albert TW Simeons. It can reduce the weight immediately and you will be able to see the change the next day.

The "Steak Day" plan is very simple: eat nothing for breakfast and lunch.

Drink a lot of water. You can also drink coffee and tea, as long as they are sugar-free. During dinner, eat a large steak. The steak can be cooked in oil or butter. You can also eat a raw apple or tomato.

Some prefer to have "Steak and Cheese Day" instead of the regular "Steak and

Cheese Day". This can also lose 2 pounds overnight. The diet plan is also very simple:

- Eat 2 eggs for breakfast.

- You can eat a large steak for lunch and dinner.

- After eating the steak, you can eat the cheese.

- Don't forget to drink plenty of water.

Always remember that "Steak Day" should be done on the same day that you notice an increase or decrease in your weight.

Effects of the HCG diet plan

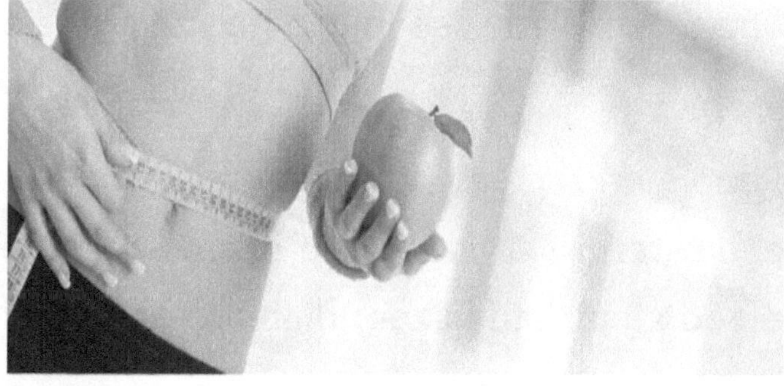

The HCG diet plan has been one of the most successful and most recommended diet programs in the world. The results are visible in a short period of time. Here are some of the positive side effects of the plan:

- Rapid weight loss, especially fat loss, for both men and women is the most important effect of this program.

- Total body transformation due to weight loss.

- Increased self-confidence.

- The metabolism rate became faster.

- Obesity can be avoided.

- The craving for sweets has decreased.

- There is a decrease in the flabby areas of the body.

- People on the HCG diet have the lowest cholesterol and stabilized blood pressure. The blood sugar stabilizes; diabetic people on the diet enjoy fewer medications.

- People become more energetic. o People are well hydrated. o There is a decrease in the symptoms of chronic disease and all forms of arthritis.

- Reduces the risk of breast cancer.

- Migraines subside and people get better sleep pattern.

Conclusion

This book has given you all the details you need to know to start an HGC diet. Divided into the different stages, you can clearly see what you need to do to maintain this diet. It will also help you see all the fruits and vegetables that you are allowed on this diet, but keep in mind that they should be eaten individually. I hope these books have been able to help you learn more about the HCG diet, specifically the four stages you need to go through.

The next step after successfully completing this set is to follow the tips provided in the books, as well as make your HCG diet a pleasant journey by trying the recipes there.

Remember that you need to follow this diet for at least three weeks to properly restore the brain. Make sure you don't exceed 42 days. If you have even more weight to lose after staying on the plan for 42 days, take the next six weeks as a break from the HCG diet.

Eat normally during the break, but try to exclude processed starches and sugars. After the break period, you can restart the diet for three to six weeks.

By rereading the book, you will be able to memorize what you need to know about the foods you can eat, and with its simple layout, you should also be able to find information at your fingertips whenever you need it.

Remember this isn't just a diet. It is a way to keep the weight off forever. As a precaution, those following any type of diet should seek the advice of their physician before starting, to ensure that the diet can be used safely with all medications that may be taken.

One more thing: can I ask you one last question?

www.ingramcontent.com/pod-product-compliance
Lightning Source LLC
Chambersburg PA
CBHW031422250726
48656CB00002B/793